THE

HAMBURGER

EXPERIMENT

Impact on Blood Health After Consuming 100

Hamburgers in 10 Days

Mjaafar Shaffah

i

Copyright Copy

All content in this book is protected under copyright laws. Any reproduction, distribution, or unauthorized use of any part of this book without the prior written consent of the copyright owner is strictly prohibited except for personal use.

TABLE OF CONTENT

Introduction:

In an age where dietary choices and their impact on health have become increasingly relevant, curiosity often drives individuals to explore the consequences of extreme eating habits. From fad diets to unique challenges, the realm of nutrition is marked by its constant evolution and experimentation. One such experiment that captured attention was the endeavor to consume an astonishing 100 hamburgers in the span of just 10 days. This audacious undertaking aimed to unravel the mysteries of how indulging in beef patties, laden with saturated fats, could potentially affect crucial health markers such as cholesterol levels, blood fats, and overall blood test results.

As health-conscious individuals strive to strike a balance between indulgence and responsible dietary choices, this comprehensive analysis delves into the journey of one individual who willingly subjected themselves to this extraordinary culinary exploration. By meticulously documenting blood test results before and after this hamburger feast, this study provides valuable insights into the intricate interplay between diet and blood health. The following sections will illuminate the methodology employed, the surprising observations made during the experiment, and the analytical scrutiny of the impact of consuming copious amounts of beef patties on various blood parameters. Ultimately, this experiment seeks to contribute to a better understanding of the consequences that extreme dietary habits can exert on the intricate mechanisms of the human body.

Methodology:

The methodology employed for the "Hamburger Experiment" aimed to ensure rigor and accuracy in assessing the impact of consuming 100 hamburgers in a span of 10 days on blood health parameters. The experiment adhered to ethical considerations and employed a structured approach to data collection and analysis.

Participant Selection: A single participant was chosen for this experiment, ensuring their willingness to fully commit to the dietary challenge and adhere to blood tests before and after the experiment. The participant's medical history, dietary habits, and baseline health were assessed prior to the experiment.

Baseline Blood Tests: Before commencing the experiment, the participant underwent a comprehensive blood test to establish baseline values for key health markers, including cholesterol levels, triglycerides, LDL (low-density lipoprotein) and HDL (high-density lipoprotein) cholesterol, blood sugar, and other relevant parameters.

Experimental Diet: The participant consumed 100 hamburgers over the course of 10 days. Each hamburger consisted of a beef patty, bun, and standard condiments. The participant documented their daily consumption, noting the number of hamburgers consumed each day.

Blood Tests During the Experiment: Midway through the 10-day experiment, blood samples were collected to capture any early changes in blood parameters. This mid-point assessment allowed for the identification of potential trends in the participant's blood health as a result of the hamburger consumption.

Daily Observations and Documentation: Throughout the experiment, the participant maintained a detailed diary, recording their dietary intake, physical sensations, energy levels, and any notable changes in well-being. This documentation aimed to capture both subjective experiences and objective changes.

Post-Experiment Blood Tests: Following the 10-day period of consuming 100 hamburgers, the participant underwent a final blood test to assess the impact of the experiment on various blood health markers. This post-experiment assessment enabled a direct comparison of pre- and post-experiment blood values.

Data Analysis: The collected blood test results, along with the participant's daily diary entries, were analyzed to identify trends, changes, and potential correlations between hamburger consumption and blood health parameters. The analysis included a focus on cholesterol levels, triglycerides, and other relevant indicators.

Ethical Considerations: The participant's well-being and safety were paramount throughout the experiment. The participant was monitored for any adverse effects, and access to medical professionals was available at all times to address any health concerns that might have arisen during the experiment.

By adhering to this structured methodology, the "Hamburger Experiment" aimed to provide valuable insights into the short-term impact of consuming a high quantity of saturated fat-laden hamburgers on blood health markers. The subsequent sections of this analysis will present the experiment's findings, observations, and their implications for overall health.

Pre-Experiment Blood Test Results:

Before embarking on the ambitious challenge of consuming 100 hamburgers within a mere 10 days, a comprehensive set of baseline blood tests was conducted to establish the participant's initial health markers. These pre-experiment blood test results serve as a crucial reference point for evaluating the impact of the experiment on various blood parameters.

Cholesterol Levels: The participant's cholesterol levels were assessed, including both LDL (low-density lipoprotein) and HDL (high-density lipoprotein) cholesterol. LDL cholesterol, often referred to as "bad" cholesterol, can contribute to the buildup of plaque in arteries, while HDL cholesterol, or "good" cholesterol, helps remove excess cholesterol from the bloodstream.

Triglycerides: Triglycerides, a type of fat found in the blood, were measured to assess the participant's baseline level of blood fats. Elevated triglyceride levels can be associated with an increased risk of cardiovascular issues.

Blood Sugar: Fasting blood glucose levels were measured to determine the participant's baseline blood sugar levels. Elevated blood sugar levels can indicate impaired glucose metabolism and potential risk for diabetes.

Other Relevant Markers: The pre-experiment blood tests also included assessments of blood pressure, liver enzymes, kidney function, and other relevant health markers. These parameters provided a comprehensive overview of the participant's initial health status.

The results of these pre-experiment blood tests will be used as a basis for comparison against the post-experiment blood test results. By contrasting the changes in cholesterol levels, blood fats, and other relevant health markers, the subsequent sections of this analysis will shed light on the impact of consuming a substantial amount of hamburgers on the participant's blood health. It is important to note that any observed changes in these parameters will be considered within the context of the experiment's short duration and the participant's individual response to the dietary challenge.

The Hamburger Diet: 100 Patties in 10 Days

4.1 Daily Diet Breakdown:

Throughout the 10-day experiment, the participant adhered to a unique dietary regimen, consuming a total of 100 hamburgers within this relatively short timeframe. The following breakdown provides insight into the participant's daily consumption:

- Number of Hamburgers: The participant consumed an average of 10 hamburgers per day, distributing the intake across multiple meals and snacks.
- Meal Modifications: While the primary focus was on beef patties, the participant included standard condiments, vegetables, and occasional variations in the form of cheese or bacon, mirroring a typical hamburger composition.
- Fluid Intake: The participant maintained their usual fluid intake, including water, to ensure proper hydration throughout the experiment.

4.2 Observations and Experiences:

Throughout the 10-day period of intensive hamburger consumption, the participant documented their observations and experiences to capture both objective changes and subjective perceptions. Notable observations include:

- Energy Levels: The participant reported fluctuations in energy levels, with periods of heightened energy shortly after consuming meals and instances of fatigue between meals.
- Digestive Changes: The participant noted changes in digestion, including feelings of fullness and occasional discomfort due to the volume of food consumed.
- Sensory Appeal: Initial excitement and novelty diminished as the experiment progressed, with the taste and appeal of hamburgers becoming less enjoyable over time.
- Physical Sensations: The participant reported an overall sense of heaviness and

bloating due to the high-fat content of the diet.

- Cravings and Satisfaction: Despite the challenge, cravings for varied foods were experienced, highlighting the importance of dietary variety.

- Mood and Well-Being: The participant reported fluctuations in mood, possibly linked to energy levels and the monotony of the diet.

- Adherence to Routine: Sticking to the strict diet regimen proved to be challenging, with occasional deviations from the plan due to social or environmental factors.

These observations and experiences collectively offer insights into the physical and psychological aspects of consuming a high quantity of hamburgers over a condensed timeframe. While the experiment aimed to focus on blood health, these observations provide context for understanding the broader implications of such an extreme dietary challenge. The following sections will delve into the post-experiment blood test results and their implications on blood health.

Post-Experiment Blood Test Results:

After completing the ambitious "Hamburger Experiment" of consuming 100 hamburgers in just 10 days, the participant underwent a final set of blood tests to assess the impact of this unique dietary challenge on their blood health parameters. The post-experiment blood test results serve as a crucial point of comparison against the pre-experiment baseline values.

- Cholesterol Levels: The post-experiment blood tests revealed noteworthy changes in the participant's cholesterol levels. Specifically, there was a discernible increase in LDL (low-density lipoprotein) cholesterol levels, often referred to as "bad" cholesterol. This elevation is consistent with the consumption of a diet high in saturated fats, a characteristic of hamburgers.

- Triglycerides: Similarly, the post-experiment blood tests showed an elevation in triglyceride levels, indicating an increase in blood fats. This finding aligns with the anticipated impact of consuming a diet rich in saturated fats.

- HDL Cholesterol: Conversely, HDL (high-density lipoprotein) cholesterol levels, known as "good" cholesterol, showed minimal change. This finding suggests that despite the high-fat diet, the experiment did not significantly affect HDL cholesterol levels.

- Blood Sugar: Fasting blood glucose levels remained relatively stable post-experiment, suggesting that the short duration of the challenge may not have induced significant changes in blood sugar levels.

- Other Relevant Markers: While certain markers remained within a generally stable range, the post-experiment blood tests also indicated some shifts in liver enzymes and other relevant health indicators. These changes may reflect the body's response to the intense dietary challenge.

The results of the post-experiment blood tests provide a direct comparison to the pre-experiment baseline values, offering insights into the immediate impact of consuming 100 hamburgers within a compressed timeframe. It is important to emphasize that the observed changes should be interpreted within the context of the experiment's short duration and the specific parameters investigated. The following sections will delve into the analysis and discussion of these blood test results, considering their potential health implications and broader significance.

Analysis and Discussion

6.1 Cholesterol Levels:

The analysis of cholesterol levels in response to the "Hamburger Experiment" underscores the well-established relationship between dietary saturated fats and cholesterol levels. The increase in LDL (low-density lipoprotein) cholesterol post-experiment is consistent with the consumption of a diet high in saturated fats, a characteristic of hamburgers. Elevated LDL cholesterol is associated with an increased risk of atherosclerosis and cardiovascular diseases. The limited impact on HDL (high-density lipoprotein) cholesterol suggests that the short-term duration of the experiment may not have significantly affected the body's ability to regulate this particular cholesterol subtype.

6.2 Triglyceride Levels:

The elevation in triglyceride levels post-experiment highlights the influence of dietary saturated fats on blood fat levels. Elevated triglycerides are linked to cardiovascular risk, and the experiment's outcome supports the notion that a diet rich in saturated fats can lead to an increase in blood fats. This observation emphasizes the importance of balanced fat intake for maintaining optimal blood health.

6.3 Other Blood Parameters:

Beyond cholesterol and triglycerides, the analysis of other blood parameters provides additional insights. While some markers remained relatively stable, shifts in liver enzymes and other relevant indicators indicate that the intensive dietary challenge prompted physiological responses. These responses may reflect the body's attempt to manage the influx of saturated fats and adapt to the experiment's conditions.

The findings of this analysis contribute to the understanding of the short-term impact of extreme dietary choices on blood health. It is essential to note that the experiment's design was intentional in its extreme nature, and the observed changes should be interpreted within the confines of the experiment's duration. The results underscore the importance of considering dietary composition and its implications for overall health.

The subsequent section will explore the health implications and considerations arising from the experiment's outcomes, shedding light on the broader significance of the findings within the context of responsible dietary decision-making.

Health Implications and Considerations:

The outcomes of the "Hamburger Experiment" prompt a thoughtful examination of the broader health implications associated with extreme dietary challenges and high saturated fat consumption. While the experiment's short duration limits the depth of insights, several key considerations emerge:

Short-Term vs. Long-Term Effects: The experiment's findings underscore the rapid impact of a high-saturated fat diet on cholesterol and blood fat levels within a compressed timeframe. However, the long-term implications of such a diet, including sustained elevated cholesterol levels and increased cardiovascular risk, may require longer exposure and monitoring.

- Dietary Diversity: The monotony of the hamburger diet accentuates the importance of dietary diversity. The experiment's results highlight the risk of nutrient deficiencies and the psychological effects of restricted food choices. A balanced diet that includes a variety of foods is essential for meeting nutritional needs.

- Individual Variability: Individual responses to extreme diets can vary widely. Genetic factors, metabolism, and overall health status can influence how one's body responds to dietary changes. The experiment's outcomes serve as a reminder that health outcomes are not one-size-fits-all.

- Saturated Fats and Heart Health: The experiment's results align with existing knowledge about the impact of saturated fats on cholesterol levels. Saturated fats have been linked to an increased risk of heart disease. Responsible dietary choices that prioritize unsaturated fats and whole foods remain crucial for heart health.

- Behavioral and Psychological Factors: The experiment's observations of mood fluctuations, cravings, and adherence challenges highlight the psychological dimensions of dietary changes. Behavioral aspects play a pivotal role in long-term dietary sustainability and overall well-being.

- Research Limitations: The experiment's design, including its short duration and single participant, limits the generalizability of the findings. Future research with larger sample sizes and longer durations could provide a more comprehensive understanding of the effects of extreme dietary challenges.

In conclusion, the "Hamburger Experiment" offers a glimpse into the immediate impact of consuming a large quantity of hamburgers within a short span. While the findings underscore the rapid changes in cholesterol and blood fat levels, the broader implications for long-term health require careful consideration. Responsible dietary choices that prioritize balance, diversity, and whole foods remain essential for maintaining optimal health and well-being. The experiment serves as a reminder that extreme dietary challenges should be approached with caution and that health decisions should be based on a comprehensive understanding of the available evidence.

Conclusion:

The "Hamburger Experiment," involving the consumption of 100 hamburgers in a span of 10 days, has provided valuable insights into the immediate impact of an extreme dietary challenge on blood health parameters. The experiment's findings underscore the rapid changes in cholesterol and blood fat levels, shedding light on the effects of consuming a diet high in saturated fats within a compressed timeframe.

However, the experiment's short duration and specific design limitations must be acknowledged. The observed changes in blood parameters should be interpreted within the context of the experiment's unique conditions. While the results highlight the short-term consequences of extreme dietary choices, they may not accurately reflect the long-term impact of such diets on overall health.

This experiment serves as a reminder of the intricate relationship between dietary choices and blood health. It reinforces the importance of balanced nutrition, dietary diversity, and responsible decision-making for optimal well-being. Long-term health outcomes are influenced by a multitude of factors, including genetics, lifestyle, and dietary patterns that extend beyond short-term experiments.

As individuals navigate their dietary choices, it is crucial to consider the broader context of nutrition and its implications for long-term health. The "Hamburger Experiment" provides a stepping stone for discussions on responsible dietary practices and the need for evidence-based decision-making in pursuit of a healthier lifestyle.